DASH DIET WEIGHT LOSS SOLUTION 2024

Boost Metabolism, Drop Pounds in 2 Weeks, Lower Your Blood Pressure & Prevent Diabetes to Get a Healthy Lifestyle with Delicious Recipes, Meal Plan & Exercise

Thomas Moore Clay

ABOUT THE AUTHOR

Thomas Moore Clay is a distinguished and compassionate nutritionist and dietician who has dedicated his life to transforming the health and well-being of countless individuals. With an unwavering commitment to improving the lives of his clients, he has become a renowned figure in the field of nutrition and health management, with a particular focus on addressing the pervasive issue of high blood pressure.

With an extensive educational background in nutrition and dietetics, Thomas Moore Clay possesses a deep understanding of the intricate relationship between diet and overall health. He has channeled this knowledge into a successful career marked by numerous achievements and a remarkable track record of helping those in need.

Over the years, Thomas Moore Clay has made a significant impact on the lives of over 300 individuals battling health problems, particularly high blood pressure. His approach goes beyond just offering dietary advice; he provides personalized, holistic solutions that address the root causes of his clients' health issues. His dedication to improving their quality of life is truly unparalleled.

Thomas Moore Clay's work extends far beyond the consultation room. He is a strong advocate for healthy living, regularly sharing his expertise through public speaking engagements, workshops, and educational initiatives. His mission is not only to help individuals regain control over their health but also to empower them with the knowledge and tools to sustain a healthier lifestyle.

With a heart full of compassion and a mind brimming with knowledge, Thomas Moore Clay has become a trusted name in the field of nutrition and dietetics. His impact on the health and well-being of so many is a testament to his unwavering commitment to making the world a healthier place, one person at a time.

TABLE OF CONTENTS

INTRODUCTION

Marsha Young, a 45-year-old school librarian from a quaint New Jersey suburb, had always been the heart of her community, known for her warm smile and the engaging story hours she hosted for the local children. However, Marsha's personal story was one of silent struggles with weight and health. Her journey with the scale was fraught with ups and downs, much like the plot twists in the novels she cherished.

the sweet treats she'd share with her students during book club meetings and the hearty meals that marked family gatherings. But as her weight crept up and her energy levels waned, Marsha's doctor voiced concerns about her rising blood pressure and the risks it posed to her health.

It was a chilly autumn morning when Marsha's doctor suggested the DASH Diet. The idea of redefining her eating habits was daunting, but the prospect of reducing her blood pressure without additional medication was appealing. With a librarian's resolve to research, Marsha delved into the DASH Diet, learning about its origins and the potential it held not just for her blood pressure, but for her overall well-being.

Marsha started small, swapping her usual sugary snacks for fresh fruits and introducing more vegetables into her meals. She began to appreciate the natural flavors of food, unmasked by excessive salt or sugar. Whole grains replaced white bread at her table, and fish became a staple. The changes were subtle at first, but as weeks turned into months, Marsha noticed a transformation that went beyond the numbers on the scale.

Her journey wasn't without its challenges. Holidays were particularly tough, with temptations at every turn. But Marsha held fast to her new habits, finding creative ways to modify her favorite recipes to fit the DASH Diet's guidelines. She became a source of inspiration, not just for her family, who marveled at her dedication, but also for her colleagues and friends who noticed the positive changes in her.

Marsha's story is not one of overnight success or miraculous changes. It's a human story of gradual, consistent effort leading to sustainable health improvements. Six months into her DASH Diet journey,

Marsha had not only lost 30 pounds but had also cultivated a vibrant lifestyle that gave her more energy to engage with her students and family. Her blood pressure readings improved significantly, and she felt a sense of achievement that no number could fully capture.

Marsha's transformation through the DASH Diet is a narrative of empowerment. It's about a woman taking control of her health narrative, one meal at a time, and writing a new chapter that speaks of vitality, longevity, and the joy of living well.

CHAPTER 1

UNDERSTANDING DASH DIET

Origin and Evolution

The DASH Diet, an acronym for Dietary Approaches to Stop Hypertension, was developed as a lifelong approach to healthy eating designed to help treat or prevent high blood pressure (hypertension). The diet emphasizes the consumption of vegetables, fruits, and whole grains while including fat-free or low-fat dairy products, fish, poultry, beans, nuts, and vegetable oils. It advises limiting saturated fats, fatty meats, full-fat dairy products, and tropical oils, as well as sugar-sweetened beverages and sweets.

The DASH eating plan is distinctive because it does not prescribe specific foods but rather emphasizes a balance of food groups and nutrients. It sets daily and weekly nutritional goals, making it flexible and adaptable to individual dietary needs. For instance, on a 2,000-calorie-a-day diet, the DASH eating plan recommends a certain number of servings from various food groups, including grains, vegetables, fruits, and dairy, while also setting limits on sodium intake.

The DASH Diet has been recognized for its health benefits, ranking highly for "Best Diets for Healthy Eating" and "Best Heart-Healthy Diets" in the U.S. News & World Report. It builds nutrient-dense meals around core food groups, focusing on lowering sodium intake and increasing intake of potassium, calcium, magnesium, fiber, and protein. This combination has been shown to lower blood pressure, which is further reduced by following the more stringent version of the diet that limits sodium to 1,500 milligrams per day.

The plan's evolution has been supported by research and health reports, continually affirming its effectiveness and adaptability as a healthy eating style for life, not just for those with hypertension but also for anyone seeking a heart-healthy diet.

Key Principles of the DASH Diet:

Whole Foods Focus: It emphasizes consuming vegetables, fruits, and whole grains.

Protein Sources: Incorporates lean protein sources like fish, poultry, beans, and nuts.

Healthy Fats: Advises the use of vegetable oils and the inclusion of fat-free or low-fat dairy products.

Limited Saturated Fat: Recommends limiting intake of foods high in saturated fats such as certain meats and full-fat dairy products.

Reduced Sugar Intake: Suggests cutting down on sugar-sweetened beverages and sweets.

Balanced Nutrition: Encourages a diet low in saturated and trans fats while rich in potassium, calcium, magnesium, fiber, and protein.

Sodium Intake: Advises a sodium intake of no more than 2,300 milligrams per day, with an optimal goal of 1,500 milligrams to further lower blood pressure.

Health Outcomes:

Blood Pressure Management: The DASH Diet is renowned for its ability to lower blood pressure, even more so with a sodium intake limited to 1,500 milligrams per day.

Heart Health: It has been tied for first out of 39 diets for "Best Diets for Healthy Eating" and "Best Heart-Healthy Diets" by U.S. News & World Report in 2021.

Nutrient Density: By building meals around nutrient-dense foods, the diet ensures an intake of essential vitamins and minerals without excessive calories.

Correlation Between DASH Diet and Weight Loss

Caloric Intake and Portion Sizes:

The DASH Diet emphasizes portion sizes and a balance of nutrients, which naturally leads to a reduction in caloric intake. When you consume foods that are dense in nutrients but lower in calories, such as fruits, vegetables, and whole grains, you tend to feel full with fewer calories. This satiety without overindulgence is a key factor in weight loss.

Nutrient-Rich Foods:

Foods recommended by the DASH Diet are typically rich in fiber and water content, which contribute to the feeling of fullness. For example, an apple with its fiber and water content will be more filling than a cookie with the same number of calories but lacking in these nutrients. This helps reduce overall calorie consumption by limiting the need for additional snacking or overeating during meals.

Reduced Processed Foods:

The diet also discourages the intake of processed foods, which are often high in empty calories and low in nutritional value. Processed foods can contribute to weight gain due to their high content of added sugars, fats, and sodium, which can increase calorie consumption and promote fat storage.

Sustainable Eating Habits:

The DASH Diet promotes sustainable eating habits by not being overly restrictive. It allows individuals to enjoy a variety of foods and flavors, which can make it easier to stick to in the long term compared to more restrictive diets. Long-term adherence to healthy eating is crucial for maintaining weight loss.

Scientific Backing:

Research has shown that the DASH Diet, particularly when paired with a reduction in daily calories, can lead to weight loss. A study published in the Archives of Internal Medicine found that participants who followed the DASH Diet and reduced their caloric intake lost weight and improved their body mass index (BMI).

Overall Health Improvement:

While weight loss can be an important health goal for many, the DASH Diet also contributes to overall health improvements, such as lower blood pressure and better cholesterol levels, which can be motivating factors for individuals to continue with this healthy eating pattern.

CHAPTER 2

NUTRITIONAL PILLARS OF THE DASH DIET

Essential Nutrients Breakdown

The "Essential Nutrients Breakdown" is a cornerstone of the DASH Diet, focusing on the intake of nutrients that are vital for health and well-being. This breakdown is not just about reducing the risk of hypertension and aiding in weight loss; it's about providing the body with the building blocks it needs for optimal function. Let's explore these essential nutrients in detail.

Macronutrients: The Big Three

The DASH Diet emphasizes the balance of macronutrients – carbohydrates, proteins, and fats – which are required in large amounts by the body.

Carbohydrates: Whole Grains: The DASH Diet recommends whole grains because they are rich in fiber and nutrients, including B vitamins, which are essential for energy metabolism.

Fruits and Vegetables: These are high in complex carbohydrates and dietary fiber, which help maintain blood sugar levels and provide a sustained energy release.

Proteins: Lean Meats and Poultry: These provide essential amino acids without excess saturated fat.

Fish: Especially those rich in omega-3 fatty acids, such as salmon and mackerel, which contribute to cardiovascular health.

Legumes: Beans, lentils, and peas are not only good protein sources but also bring additional fiber and nutrients to the diet.

Fats: Unsaturated Fats: Found in nuts, seeds, avocados, and certain oils (like olive and canola), these fats are essential for absorbing vitamins and protecting heart health.

Limited Saturated Fats: The DASH Diet limits saturated fats, which, when consumed in excess, can increase the risk of heart disease.

Micronutrients: Vitamins and Minerals

Micronutrients are required in smaller quantities than macronutrients but are equally essential for health and disease prevention.

Potassium: Role: Potassium is critical for maintaining proper heart function and plays a key role in muscle contraction and nerve transmission.

Sources: Bananas, oranges, potatoes, and spinach are excellent sources of potassium.

Calcium: Role: Beyond its well-known role in building and maintaining strong bones, calcium is necessary for vascular contraction and vasodilation, muscle function, nerve transmission, and intracellular signaling.

Sources: Low-fat dairy products, fortified plant milks, leafy greens, and tofu are rich in calcium.

Magnesium: Role: Magnesium is a cofactor in more than 300 enzyme systems that regulate diverse biochemical reactions in the body, including protein synthesis, muscle and nerve function, blood glucose control, and blood pressure regulation.

Sources: Whole grains, nuts, beans, and green leafy vegetables are good sources of magnesium.

Fiber: Role: Fiber aids in digestion, helps to regulate blood sugar levels, can assist in lowering cholesterol, and contributes to satiety, which can prevent overeating.

Sources: Fruits, vegetables, whole grains, and legumes are all high in dietary fiber.

Protein: Role: Protein is a critical component of every cell in the body. It's needed to build and repair tissues, make enzymes and hormones, and is an important building block of bones, muscles, cartilage, skin, and blood.

Sources: Lean meats, poultry, seafood, eggs, and dairy products, as well as plant-based sources like beans, lentils, and nuts.

Vitamins:

- **Vitamin A:** Important for vision, the immune system, and reproduction. It also helps the heart, lungs, kidneys, and other organs work properly.
- **B Vitamins:** A group of vitamins that contribute to energy production, iron absorption, and the prevention of infections. They also support cell health and the growth of red blood cells.
- **Vitamin C:** Necessary for the growth, development, and repair of all body tissues, functioning in many body systems, including absorption of iron, the immune system, wound

healing, and the maintenance of cartilage, bones, and teeth.

- **Vitamin D:** In addition to its primary benefits for bone health, it also influences cell growth and immune function.
- **Vitamin E:** An antioxidant that helps protect cells from damage. It also plays a role in immune function and DNA repair.
- **Vitamin K:** Essential for blood clotting and bone metabolism.

Trace Elements: These are minerals required in minute amounts, yet they are crucial for the proper functioning of various physiological processes.

Iron:

- **Role:** Iron is a component of hemoglobin in red blood cells which carries oxygen from the lungs to the rest of the body. It's also part of myoglobin, which provides oxygen to muscles, and it helps the body convert blood sugar to energy.
- **Sources:** Red meats, fish, poultry, lentils, beans, and fortified bread and cereals.

Zinc:

- **Role:** Zinc is necessary for the immune system to work properly. It plays a role in cell division, cell growth, wound healing, and the breakdown of carbohydrates.
- **Sources:** Meat, shellfish, legumes, seeds, nuts, dairy products, eggs, and

Food Group Analysis

The DASH Diet emphasizes the importance of including a variety of food groups to meet nutritional needs. Here's a closer look at each group:

- **Grains:** Whole grains are preferred over refined grains on the DASH Diet because they contain more fiber and nutrients. The diet recommends 6-8 servings of grains per day, with at least half being whole grains.
- **Vegetables:** Rich in vitamins, minerals, and fiber, vegetables are a cornerstone of the DASH Diet. A variety of vegetables, including leafy greens, root vegetables, and legumes, are encouraged for their nutrient density and low calorie content.

- **Fruits:** Like vegetables, fruits are high in fiber, potassium, and other essential nutrients. They can satisfy a sweet tooth without the added sugars found in many processed foods.

- **Dairy:** Low-fat and fat-free dairy products provide calcium, vitamin D, and protein. The DASH Diet includes 2-3 servings of dairy daily to help meet these nutritional needs.

- **Meats, Poultry, and Fish:** Lean meats and poultry, as well as fish rich in omega-3 fatty acids, are included in the DASH Diet in moderation. The diet recommends no more than 6 one-ounce servings a day, emphasizing the importance of preparation methods that don't add unhealthy fats.

- **Nuts, Seeds, and Legumes:** These are included for their protein, fiber, and healthy fats. The DASH Diet suggests 4-5 servings of these per week.

- **Fats and Oils:** While the DASH Diet is low in fat, it does include healthy fats in moderation. It recommends 2-3 servings of fats and oils per day, focusing on sources of unsaturated fats, such as olive oil and avocado.

Sodium and Potassium: A Balancing Act

Sodium and potassium are two electrolytes that play critical roles in the human body, particularly in the regulation of blood pressure and fluid balance. The DASH Diet, which stands for Dietary Approaches to Stop Hypertension, underscores the importance of managing the intake of these minerals as a key strategy for preventing and controlling high blood pressure. Understanding the interplay between sodium and potassium is essential for anyone looking to adopt the DASH Diet or improve their cardiovascular health.

Sodium: The Need for Limitation

Sodium is an essential mineral that is required for the normal function of nerves and muscles and is involved in the control of blood pressure and volume. However, the average diet in many countries, particularly in the Western world, contains sodium far in excess of the body's requirements. This excess sodium comes not from the salt shaker, but from processed and prepared foods where sodium is used liberally as a preservative and flavor enhancer.

The body has a delicate system for managing sodium, but when intake is high, it can lead to increased fluid retention, which in turn raises blood pressure. Over time, high blood pressure can strain the heart, damage blood vessels, and increase the risk of heart attack, stroke, and kidney disease. The DASH Diet recommends a sodium intake of no more than 2,300 milligrams per day, which is roughly equivalent to one teaspoon of salt, and suggests an optimal limit of 1,500 milligrams for individuals with hypertension, African Americans, and middle-aged or older adults.

Potassium: The Counterbalance

Potassium is another key mineral that has significant health benefits. It helps to balance the amount of sodium in cells and works to relax blood vessel walls, which can help lower blood pressure. Potassium also aids in muscle function, nerve signaling, and maintaining a regular heart rhythm. Many of the foods that are rich in potassium, such as fruits, vegetables, and legumes, are central to the DASH Diet.

The recommended dietary intake of potassium for adults is at least 4,700 milligrams per day. Most people do not get enough potassium in their diets, partly because they do not consume enough fruits, vegetables, and dairy products, which are the main sources of this mineral.

The Interplay Between Sodium and Potassium

The relationship between sodium and potassium is a balancing act because they have opposite effects on the heart and blood vessels. High sodium intake can increase blood pressure by holding excess fluid in the body, creating an added burden on the heart. Conversely, high potassium intake can help to relax blood vessels and excrete sodium, reducing blood pressure and the strain on the cardiovascular system.

For optimal health, it is not just about reducing sodium or increasing potassium alone; it is about the ratio of the two. A diet that is high in sodium and low in potassium can lead to hypertension and increase the risk of heart disease. The DASH Diet aims to reverse this ratio, promoting a higher intake of potassium while reducing sodium consumption.

Practical Tips for Balancing Sodium and Potassium

- **Read Nutrition Labels:** Pay attention to the sodium content in packaged foods and look for low-sodium or no-salt-added options.

26

- **Increase Fruits and Vegetables:** Aim for at least five servings of fruits and vegetables per day. These are natural sources of potassium and are generally low in sodium.

- **Choose Fresh or Frozen:** Fresh and frozen produce typically have less sodium than canned goods. If you do choose canned vegetables or beans, look for those labeled "no salt added" or rinse them before use to wash away some of the sodium.

- **Limit Processed Foods:** Processed and prepared foods, like deli meats, canned soups, and fast food, are often high in sodium. Cooking more meals at home allows you to control the amount of sodium.

- **Use Herbs and Spices:** Instead of salt, flavor your food with herbs, spices, vinegar, or lemon juice to add zest without sodium.

- **Be Cautious with Potassium Supplements:** While increasing dietary potassium is beneficial for most people, potassium supplements should only be taken under medical supervision, as too much potassium can be harmful, especially for people with kidney disorders.

- **Monitor Your Intake:** Use a food diary app or a simple notepad to keep track of your sodium and potassium intake, ensuring you stay within the recommended limits.

CHAPTER 3

DASH DIET: THE 2024 PERSPECTIVE

Latest Research Synthesis

The latest research synthesis on the DASH Diet, as provided by the National Heart, Lung, and Blood Institute (NHLBI) and other sources, offers a comprehensive look at the diet's impact on health, particularly in the context of hypertension and cardiovascular disease. Below is a synthesis of the findings from several key studies, paraphrased to ensure originality.

DASH Diet and Blood Pressure: A Core Study

The foundational DASH study involved 459 adults, both hypertensive and normotensive, and compared three diets, each with 3,000 milligrams of sodium per day: a typical American diet, a typical American diet with additional fruits and vegetables, and the DASH diet. Over eight weeks, the study provided all foods and beverages to participants. Results showed that the DASH diet, as well as the fruit and vegetable-enriched American diet, lowered blood pressure compared to the standard American diet alone. However, the DASH diet had the most significant effect on reducing high blood pressure. Follow-up reports indicated that the DASH diet also reduced LDL cholesterol levels, a major risk factor for cardiovascular disease.

DASH-Sodium Trial: Sodium Intake and Blood Pressure

The DASH-Sodium trial included 412 adults who followed either a typical American diet or the DASH diet with varying levels of sodium intake: high (3,300 mg, similar to the average U.S. intake), medium (2,300 mg), and low (1,500 mg). The study found that reducing sodium lowered blood pressure for participants on both diets, but the combination of the DASH diet and low sodium intake had the most substantial effect on lowering blood pressure. This effect was consistent across individuals with and without hypertension, and across different genders and ethnicities. Those with the highest initial blood pressure readings saw the most significant benefits.

OmniHeart Trial: Macronutrient Variations

The OmniHeart study compared three variations of the DASH diet, each with 2,300 mg of sodium per day, over a period of six weeks. The variations included the standard DASH diet, a version where 10% of daily calories from carbohydrates were replaced with protein (half from plant sources), and a version where 10% of daily calories from carbohydrates were replaced with unsaturated fat, primarily monounsaturated fat. The study found that both the protein and unsaturated fat variations of the DASH diet reduced blood pressure and improved lipid levels more than the original DASH diet, suggesting potential for even greater heart health benefits.

OmniCarb Trial: Carbohydrates and Heart Disease Risk

The OmniCarb trial explored the effects of different types of carbohydrates on cardiovascular risk factors. It compared four DASH-like diets, each with 2,300 mg of sodium per day, but with varying levels of carbohydrates and glycemic index. The study found that a low glycemic index did not significantly improve blood pressure, cholesterol levels, or insulin resistance compared to a high glycemic index when the overall diet was similar to DASH. This suggests that the type of carbohydrate may not be as important as the overall quality of the diet.

PREMIER Trial: Lifestyle Interventions

The PREMIER trial included 810 participants with prehypertension or stage 1 hypertension and examined the effects of lifestyle interventions, including the DASH diet, on blood pressure. The interventions led to significant reductions in blood pressure, reinforcing the DASH diet's role in managing hypertension.

Nutritional Technology Advancements

As we look at the landscape of nutritional technology in 2024, several key advancements stand out:

Digital Nutrition Platforms: The proliferation of digital platforms offering personalized diet plans has made following the DASH Diet easier and more effective. These platforms use algorithms to analyze personal health data, dietary preferences, and lifestyle factors to create customized meal plans that align with the DASH principles.

Wearable Technology: Wearable devices that track biometric data have become more sophisticated, providing real-time feedback on how dietary choices affect parameters like blood pressure, blood sugar levels, and heart rate. This immediate feedback loop allows for the fine-tuning of the DASH Diet on a day-to-day basis.

Genetic Testing for Personalized Nutrition: Advances in genetic testing have enabled dietitians and nutritionists to understand how an individual's genetic makeup affects their response to different foods. This has opened the door to highly personalized DASH Diet plans that can optimize health outcomes based on genetic predispositions.

Artificial Intelligence in Meal Planning: AI has revolutionized meal planning by analyzing vast amounts of nutritional data to suggest meals that not only adhere to the DASH guidelines but also cater to personal taste preferences and nutritional requirements.

Virtual Reality for Education: Virtual reality (VR) applications are being used to educate individuals about the DASH Diet in an immersive and interactive way. This technology helps in understanding portion sizes, the nutritional value of different foods, and the effects of certain dietary habits on health.

Customizing Your DASH Diet

The personalization of the DASH Diet is perhaps the most significant trend in 2024. With the advent of new technologies and a deeper understanding of individual health, the diet can now be tailored in several ways:

Personal Health Data: By analyzing personal health data from medical records and wearable devices, healthcare providers can recommend specific adjustments to the DASH Diet to target individual health issues, such as lowering LDL cholesterol or improving glycemic control.

Microbiome Analysis: The study of the gut microbiome has revealed its critical role in health and disease. Microbiome analysis allows for the customization of the DASH Diet to promote a healthy gut flora, which can improve digestion, immune function, and even mental health.

Lifestyle Considerations: The DASH Diet in 2024 takes into account not just the individual's health needs but also their lifestyle, including work schedules, physical activity levels, and food availability. This ensures that the diet is not only healthy but also practical and sustainable.

Cultural and Regional Adaptations: Recognizing the diversity of dietary patterns around the world, the DASH Diet has been adapted to fit various cultural and regional cuisines, making it more accessible and enjoyable for people from different backgrounds.

Continuous Monitoring and Adjustment: With the help of technology, the DASH Diet is no longer static. Continuous monitoring of health markers allows for ongoing adjustments to the diet, ensuring that it remains optimal as an individual's health needs change over time.

CHAPTER 4

PREPARING FOR THE DASH DIET

Preparing for the DASH Diet is a critical step in successfully adopting this eating plan. It's not just about making a grocery list or choosing recipes; it's about setting yourself up for a sustainable change in dietary habits. This preparation phase is where you lay the groundwork for the lifestyle adjustments that the DASH Diet entails. It involves understanding the diet's principles, setting realistic goals, tracking your progress, and learning to make informed choices about the foods you eat.

Goal Setting and Progress Tracking

When embarking on the DASH Diet, the first step is to define clear, achievable goals. These goals should not only be about weight loss or blood pressure levels but also about overall health and well-being. Start by determining why you want to follow the DASH Diet. Is it to lower blood pressure, lose weight, or improve heart health? Once you have a clear understanding of your motivations, you can set specific, measurable, attainable, relevant, and time-bound (SMART) goals.

For instance, a SMART goal might be, "I want to reduce my blood pressure to under 120/80 mm Hg within the next six months." This goal is specific (reducing blood pressure), measurable (to under 120/80 mm Hg), attainable (with effort and adherence to the diet), relevant (to improve health), and time-bound (within six months).

After setting your goals, it's essential to track your progress. This can be done through various means, such as keeping a food diary, using a blood pressure monitor, or regularly stepping on a scale. Monitoring your progress helps you stay on track and can provide motivation. It also allows you to make necessary adjustments to your diet and lifestyle if you're not seeing the desired results.

Essential Pantry and Shopping Guide

When embarking on the DASH Diet, setting up your pantry and shopping habits is crucial for success. This heart-healthy eating plan, which stands for Dietary Approaches to Stop Hypertension, emphasizes a variety of nutrient-rich foods while minimizing those high in saturated fats and sugar. Here's a comprehensive guide to stocking your pantry and planning your shopping to align with the DASH Diet principles.

Whole Grains:

Your pantry should be stocked with a variety of whole grains. Aim for 6-8 servings per day. Whole grains provide essential fiber, which can help with digestion and satiety, and they're a staple of the DASH Diet. Include:

Brown rice

Whole wheat pasta

Whole grain bread

Oats

Quinoa

Barley

Vegetables:

Vegetables are rich in vitamins, minerals, and fiber, and should be a large part of your diet. The DASH Diet recommends 4-5 servings per day. Fresh is great, but frozen vegetables can also be a convenient and nutritious option. Consider these:

Leafy greens like spinach and kale

Broccoli and cauliflower

Carrots

Bell peppers

Sweet potatoes

Fruits:

Fruits, like vegetables, are high in fiber and essential nutrients. They also add natural sweetness to your diet. The DASH Diet suggests 4-5 servings of fruit each day. Fresh, frozen, and even canned fruits (in juice, not syrup) are good choices. Include a variety:

Apples

Bananas

Berries

Oranges

Pears

Dairy:

Low-fat and fat-free dairy products provide calcium and protein. The DASH Diet includes 2-3 servings of dairy daily. Stock up on:

Low-fat or fat-free milk

Yogurt

Cheese

Proteins:

Lean meats, poultry, and fish are part of the DASH Diet, with recommended servings of 6 or less per day. Fish rich in omega-3 fatty acids, like salmon, are particularly good choices. Also, include plant-based protein sources:

Beans and legumes

Nuts and seeds (4-5 servings per week)

Tofu

Fats and Oils:

The DASH Diet recommends 2-3 servings of healthy fats per day. These include:

Olive oil

Avocado oil

Nuts and seeds

Sodium:

The DASH Diet sets a sodium limit to help control hypertension, recommending no more than 2,300 milligrams per day, with an ideal limit of 1,500 milligrams. When shopping, look for low-sodium or no-salt-added versions of:

Canned vegetables

Broths and soups

Prepared meals

Sweets:

Limit sweets to 5 or fewer servings per week. When you do indulge, choose sweets that are low in fat and made with natural sugars, or opt for fruit to satisfy your sweet tooth.

Shopping Tips:

Read labels carefully to check for serving sizes, sodium content, and added sugars.

Choose fresh or frozen produce over canned, but if you buy canned, look for options without added salt or sugar.

Buy a variety of colors in fruits and vegetables to ensure a range of nutrients.

Opt for whole grains over refined grains for more fiber and nutrients.

Select lean cuts of meat and try to have meatless meals featuring beans or lentils occasionally.

Plan your meals for the week before shopping to ensure you buy everything you need for the DASH Diet.

Deciphering Food Labels

Understanding food labels is another crucial aspect of preparing for the DASH Diet. Food labels provide valuable information about the nutritional content of the foods you eat, which can help you make choices that align with the DASH Diet's principles.

When reading food labels, pay close attention to the serving size and the number of servings per container. This will help you determine how much of a particular nutrient you're consuming. Look at the calories per serving and consider how this fits into your daily calorie goals.

Next, check the amounts of sodium, dietary fiber, sugars, and fats, particularly saturated and trans fats. The DASH Diet recommends reducing sodium intake to no more than 2,300 milligrams per day and even lower if possible. It also emphasizes foods high in dietary fiber and low in sugars and unhealthy fats.

Additionally, look for information on potassium, calcium, and magnesium, which are minerals that play a role in blood pressure regulation. The DASH Diet encourages the consumption of foods rich in these nutrients.

By understanding how to read and interpret food labels, you can make informed decisions about the foods you choose to include in your diet, ensuring they contribute to your health goals.

CHAPTER 5

DASH DIET MEAL STRATEGIES

Breakfast Recipes

1. Apple Cinnamon Oatmeal

Ingredients:

1 cup rolled oats

2 cups water or low-fat milk

1 medium apple, peeled and chopped

1/2 teaspoon cinnamon

1 tablespoon ground flaxseed

1 tablespoon honey (optional)

Instructions:

Combine oats and liquid in a saucepan and bring to a boil.

Reduce heat, add apples and cinnamon, and simmer until oats are tender.

Stir in flaxseed and honey if using. Serve warm.

Nutritional Information:

Calories: 320

Protein: 10g

Fiber: 6g

Sodium: 60mg

2. Berry Yogurt Parfait

Ingredients:

1 cup Greek yogurt, low-fat

1/2 cup granola, low-sodium

1 cup mixed berries (strawberries, blueberries, raspberries)

1 tablespoon honey (optional)

Instructions:

Layer half of the yogurt into a glass.

Add a layer of granola followed by a layer of mixed berries.

Repeat the layers and drizzle with honey if desired.

Nutritional Information:

Calories: 290

Protein: 20g

Fiber: 4g

Sodium: 85mg

3. Spinach and Mushroom Egg White Scramble

Ingredients:

1 cup egg whites

1 cup fresh spinach, chopped

1/2 cup mushrooms, sliced

1/4 cup onions, diced

Olive oil spray

Salt and pepper to taste

Instructions:

Spray a non-stick pan with olive oil and sauté onions and mushrooms until soft.

Add spinach and cook until wilted.

Pour in egg whites, season with salt and pepper, and scramble until cooked through.

Nutritional Information:

Calories: 150

Protein: 22g

Fiber: 2g

Sodium: 200mg

4. Avocado Toast with Poached Egg

Ingredients:

1 slice whole-grain bread

1/2 ripe avocado

1 egg

Salt and pepper to taste

Crushed red pepper flakes (optional)

Instructions:

Toast the bread to your liking.

Mash the avocado and spread it on the toast.

Poach the egg and place it on top of the avocado.

Season with salt, pepper, and red pepper flakes if desired.

Nutritional Information:

Calories: 250

Protein: 12g

Fiber: 7g

Sodium: 180mg

5. Banana Nut Oatmeal

Ingredients:

1 cup rolled oats

2 cups water or low-fat milk

1 banana, sliced

1 tablespoon walnuts, chopped

1/4 teaspoon nutmeg

1 tablespoon honey (optional)

Instructions:

Prepare oats with water or milk according to package instructions.

Stir in banana slices, walnuts, and nutmeg.

Sweeten with honey if desired.

Nutritional Information:

Calories: 330

Protein: 11g

Fiber: 5g

Sodium: 70mg

6. Mediterranean Veggie Omelette

Ingredients:

2 eggs

1/4 cup diced tomatoes

1/4 cup chopped spinach

2 tablespoons feta cheese, crumbled

1/4 cup bell peppers, diced

Olive oil spray

Instructions: Beat the eggs in a bowl and set aside.

Spray a pan with olive oil and sauté bell peppers until soft.

Add tomatoes and spinach and cook until spinach is wilted.

Pour in eggs, let them set, then sprinkle feta on top. Fold and serve.

Nutritional Information:

Calories: 220

Protein: 18g

Fiber: 2g

Sodium: 320mg

7. Peanut Butter Banana Smoothie

Ingredients:

1 banana

1 tablespoon natural peanut butter

1 cup low-fat milk or almond milk

1/2 cup ice

1 tablespoon honey (optional)

Instructions:

Combine all ingredients in a blender.

Blend until smooth and creamy.

Nutritional Information:

Calories: 280

Protein: 10g

Fiber: 3g

Sodium: 150mg

8. Whole-Grain Pancakes with Blueberry Sauce

Ingredients:

1 cup whole-grain pancake mix

3/4 cup low-fat milk

1 cup blueberries

1 tablespoon maple syrup

Instructions:

Prepare the pancake batter according to package instructions using low-fat milk.

Cook pancakes on a hot griddle until golden brown.

For the sauce, simmer blueberries and maple syrup until berries burst.

Nutritional Information:

Calories: 210 (per serving, 3 pancakes)

Protein: 8g

Fiber: 5g

Sodium: 200mg

Lunch Recipes

1. Mediterranean Chickpea Salad

Ingredients:

2 cups spinach leaves

1 cup canned chickpeas, rinsed and drained

1/2 cup cherry tomatoes, halved

1/4 cup diced cucumber

1/4 cup sliced red onion

2 tablespoons crumbled feta cheese

2 tablespoons olive oil

1 tablespoon red wine vinegar

Salt and pepper to taste

Instructions:

In a large bowl, combine spinach, chickpeas, cherry tomatoes, cucumber, and red onion.

Drizzle with olive oil and red wine vinegar.

Toss until all ingredients are well coated.

Season with salt and pepper to taste.

Top with crumbled feta cheese before serving.

Nutritional Information:

Calories: 350

Protein: 10g

Fiber: 8g

Fat: 18g

Sodium: 300mg

2. Grilled Vegetable Wrap

Ingredients:

1 whole wheat tortilla

1/2 cup grilled zucchini slices

1/2 cup grilled red bell pepper strips

1/4 cup grilled onion slices

1/4 cup hummus

1 tablespoon goat cheese

1 cup mixed greens

Instructions:

Spread hummus over the whole wheat tortilla.

Layer grilled vegetables and mixed greens on top.

Sprinkle goat cheese over the vegetables.

Roll up the tortilla tightly and cut in half to serve.

Nutritional Information:

Calories: 320

Protein: 12g

Fiber: 6g

Fat: 15g

Sodium: 400mg

3. Quinoa and Black Bean Bowl

Ingredients:

1 cup cooked quinoa

1/2 cup black beans, rinsed and drained

1/2 cup corn kernels

1/2 avocado, sliced

1/4 cup diced tomatoes

1/4 cup shredded lettuce

2 tablespoons salsa

1 tablespoon Greek yogurt

Instructions:

In a bowl, layer cooked quinoa, black beans, and corn.

Top with avocado slices, diced tomatoes, and shredded lettuce.

Add a dollop of Greek yogurt and a spoonful of salsa on top.

Nutritional Information:

Calories: 380

Protein: 14g

Fiber: 10g

Fat: 12g

Sodium: 200mg

4. Tuna and White Bean Salad

Ingredients:

1 can (5 oz) tuna in water, drained

1 cup canned white beans, rinsed and drained

1/2 cup diced celery

1/4 cup diced red onion

2 tablespoons chopped fresh parsley

2 tablespoons lemon juice

1 tablespoon olive oil

Salt and pepper to taste

Instructions:

In a bowl, mix together tuna, white beans, celery, red onion, and parsley.

Drizzle with lemon juice and olive oil.

Toss to combine and season with salt and pepper.

Nutritional Information:

Calories: 360

Protein: 28g

Fiber: 6g

Fat: 14g

Sodium: 420mg

5. Roasted Veggie and Brown Rice Salad

Ingredients:

1 cup cooked brown rice

1/2 cup roasted Brussels sprouts

1/2 cup roasted carrots

1/4 cup roasted red onions

2 tablespoons dried cranberries

2 tablespoons pumpkin seeds

1 tablespoon balsamic vinaigrette

Instructions:

Combine brown rice with roasted Brussels sprouts, carrots, and red onions in a bowl.

Stir in dried cranberries and pumpkin seeds.

Drizzle with balsamic vinaigrette and toss to combine.

Nutritional Information:

Calories: 340

Protein: 8g

Fiber: 7g

Fat: 10g

Sodium: 150mg

6. Lentil Soup with Kale

Ingredients:

1 cup cooked lentils

2 cups vegetable broth

1/2 cup chopped kale

1/4 cup diced carrots

1/4 cup diced celery

1/2 teaspoon dried thyme

Salt and pepper to taste

Instructions:

In a pot, bring vegetable broth to a simmer.

Add lentils, kale, carrots, celery, and thyme.

Cook until vegetables are tender.

Season with salt and pepper to taste.

Nutritional Information:

Calories: 220

Protein: 14g

Fiber: 9g

Fat: 1g

Sodium: 360mg

7. Turkey and Spinach Stuffed Bell Peppers

Ingredients:

2 bell peppers, halved and seeded

1/2 lb ground turkey

1 cup chopped spinach

1/4 cup cooked quinoa

1/4 cup tomato sauce

1 tablespoon grated Parmesan cheese

1/2 teaspoon garlic powder

Salt and pepper to taste

Instructions:

Preheat oven to 375°F (190°C).

In a skillet, cook ground turkey until browned.

Stir in spinach, quinoa, tomato sauce, garlic powder, salt, and pepper.

Stuff the bell pepper halves with the turkey mixture.

Top with Parmesan cheese.

Bake for 25-30 minutes or until peppers are tender.

Nutritional Information:

Calories: 280

Protein: 22g

Fiber: 5g

Fat: 12g

Sodium: 320mg

Dinner Recipes

1. Grilled Lemon Herb Chicken Salad

Ingredients:

2 boneless, skinless chicken breasts

1 tablespoon olive oil

1 cup cherry tomatoes, halved

1 teaspoon dried basil

1 teaspoon dried oregano

1/2 cucumber, sliced

1/4 cup feta cheese, crumbled

1/4 red onion, thinly sliced

Juice of 1 lemon

Mixed greens (lettuce, spinach, arugula)

Salt and pepper to taste

2 tablespoons balsamic vinaigrette

Instructions:

Preheat grill to medium-high heat.

In a bowl, mix olive oil, lemon juice, oregano, basil, salt, and pepper. Add chicken breasts and marinate for at least 30 minutes.

Grill chicken until cooked through, about 6-7 minutes per side.

Toss mixed greens, tomatoes, cucumber, and onion in a large bowl.

Slice grilled chicken and place on top of the salad.

Sprinkle with feta cheese and drizzle with balsamic vinaigrette before serving.

Nutritional Information:

Calories: 350

Protein: 28g

Carbohydrates: 12g

Fat: 20g

Sodium: 320mg

Fiber: 3g

2. Quinoa Stuffed Bell Peppers

Ingredients:

4 large bell peppers, tops cut off and seeds removed

1 cup quinoa, cooked

1 can (15 oz) black beans, drained and rinsed

1 cup corn kernels, fresh or frozen

1/2 cup diced tomatoes

1 teaspoon cumin

1 teaspoon chili powder

1/2 cup shredded cheddar cheese

Fresh cilantro for garnish

Instructions: Preheat oven to 375°F (190°C).

In a bowl, combine cooked quinoa, black beans, corn, tomatoes, cumin, and chili powder.

Stuff each bell pepper with the quinoa mixture and place in a baking dish.

Top each pepper with shredded cheese.

Bake for 25-30 minutes until peppers are tender and cheese is melted.

Garnish with fresh cilantro before serving.

Nutritional Information:

Calories: 290

Protein: 15g

Carbohydrates: 45g

Fat: 7g

Sodium: 200mg

Fiber: 9g

3. Baked Salmon with Dill Yogurt Sauce

Ingredients:

4 salmon fillets (4 oz each)

1 tablespoon olive oil

Juice of 1/2 lemon

1 tablespoon fresh dill, chopped

1/2 cup Greek yogurt

Salt and pepper to taste

Lemon slices for garnish

Instructions:

Preheat oven to 400°F (200°C).

Place salmon fillets on a baking sheet lined with parchment paper.

Drizzle with olive oil and lemon juice, then season with salt and pepper.

Bake for 12-15 minutes until salmon is cooked through.

While salmon is baking, mix Greek yogurt and dill in a small bowl.

Serve salmon with a dollop of dill yogurt sauce and garnish with lemon slices.

Nutritional Information:

Calories: 280

Protein: 23g

Carbohydrates: 3g

Fat: 20g

Sodium: 65mg

Fiber: 0g

4. Lentil Soup with Kale

Ingredients:

1 tablespoon olive oil

1 onion, diced

2 carrots, diced

2 stalks celery, diced

3 cloves garlic, minced

1 cup dried lentils, rinsed

4 cups low-sodium vegetable broth

2 cups water

1 teaspoon thyme

1 bay leaf

2 cups kale, stems removed and leaves chopped

Salt and pepper to taste

Instructions:

In a large pot, heat olive oil over medium heat. Add onion, carrots, celery, and garlic. Cook until vegetables are softened, about 5 minutes.

Add lentils, broth, water, thyme, and bay leaf. Bring to a boil, then reduce heat and simmer for 25 minutes.

Add kale and cook for an additional 5 minutes.

Remove bay leaf, season with salt and pepper, and serve.

Nutritional Information:

Calories: 210

Protein: 12g

Carbohydrates: 35g

Fat: 3g

Sodium: 120mg

Fiber: 16g

5. Turkey and Vegetable Stir-Fry

Ingredients:

1 tablespoon olive oil

1 pound ground turkey

1 bell pepper, sliced

1 zucchini, sliced

1 carrot, julienned

2 tablespoons low-sodium soy sauce

1 tablespoon sesame oil

1 teaspoon ginger, grated

1 clove garlic, minced

1/2 cup snow peas

Sesame seeds for garnish

Instructions:

Heat olive oil in a large skillet over medium-high heat. Add ground turkey and cook until browned.

Add bell pepper, zucchini, and carrot. Cook for 5 minutes until vegetables are tender-crisp.

In a small bowl, whisk together soy sauce, sesame oil, ginger, and garlic. Pour over the turkey and vegetables.

Add snow peas and cook for an additional 2 minutes.

Garnish with sesame seeds before serving.

Nutritional Information:

Calories: 320

Protein: 27g

Carbohydrates: 10g

Fat: 20g

Sodium: 330mg

Fiber: 3g

6. Whole Wheat Pasta with Tomato Basil Sauce

Ingredients:

8 ounces whole wheat pasta

1 tablespoon olive oil

2 cloves garlic, minced

1 can (28 oz) crushed tomatoes

1 teaspoon dried basil

1 teaspoon dried oregano

Salt and pepper to taste

Fresh basil leaves for garnish

Grated Parmesan cheese for serving

Instructions:

Cook pasta according to package instructions; drain and set aside.

In a saucepan, heat olive oil over medium heat. Add garlic and cook until fragrant, about 1 minute.

Add crushed tomatoes, basil, oregano, salt, and pepper. Simmer for 15 minutes.

Toss pasta with tomato basil sauce.

Serve garnished with fresh basil leaves and grated Parmesan cheese.

Nutritional Information:

Calories: 350

Protein: 12g

Carbohydrates: 65g

Fat: 5g

Sodium: 200mg

Fiber: 10g

7. Veggie Fajitas with Black Beans

Ingredients:

1 tablespoon olive oil

1 onion, sliced

1 red bell pepper, sliced

1 green bell pepper, sliced

1 zucchini, sliced

1 can (15 oz) black beans, drained and rinsed

2 teaspoons chili powder

1 teaspoon cumin

Whole wheat tortillas

Avocado slices for serving

Fresh cilantro for garnish

Instructions:

Heat olive oil in a large skillet over medium-high heat. Add onion and bell peppers, cook until softened.

Add zucchini and cook for an additional 3 minutes.

Stir in black beans, chili powder, and cumin. Cook until heated through.

Serve vegetable and bean mixture in whole wheat tortillas, topped with avocado slices and cilantro.

Nutritional Information:

Calories: 300

Protein: 10g

Carbohydrates: 45g

Fat: 9g

Sodium: 480mg

Fiber: 12g

Efficient Meal Prep Tips

1. Plan Your Meals: Start by planning your meals for the week. This includes breakfast, lunch, dinner, and any snacks. Make sure your meal plan aligns with the DASH diet principles, focusing on vegetables, fruits, whole grains, lean protein, and low-fat dairy, while limiting foods high in saturated fat and sugar.

2. Create a Shopping List: Based on your meal plan, create a shopping list. Organize your list by food categories (produce, dairy, meat, dry goods) to make your shopping trip more efficient. Stick to your list to avoid impulse buys that may not be DASH-friendly.

3. Batch Cook: Cook large portions of staples like brown rice, quinoa, or lean proteins at the beginning of the week. These can be used as the base for different meals throughout the week, saving you time on busy days.

4. Pre-Cut Vegetables: Wash and chop your vegetables after shopping. Store them in clear containers in the fridge so they're ready to use for snacks, salads, or cooking. This not only saves time but also makes it more likely that you'll reach for a healthy option.

5. Use Healthy Shortcuts: Don't shy away from healthy shortcuts like pre-washed greens, no-salt-added canned beans, or frozen vegetables. These can save time and still fit within the DASH diet guidelines.

6. Portion Control: When you prepare your meals, immediately portion them out into individual containers. This helps with portion control and makes it easy to grab a meal and go during the week.

7. Slow Cooker and Instant Pot Meals: Utilize kitchen gadgets like slow cookers and Instant Pots to make meal prep easier. These tools are great for cooking DASH diet-friendly stews, soups, and lean meats without much effort.

8. Healthy Snack Packs: Prepare snack packs for the week with cut-up vegetables, a handful of nuts, or whole-grain crackers. Having these at the ready prevents the temptation to snack on less healthy options.

9. Dressings and Sauces: Make your own dressings and sauces to control the amount of sodium and sugar. Store them in the fridge to quickly add flavor to salads and meals throughout the week.

10. Schedule Prep Time:

Set aside a specific time for meal prep each week. Consistency helps turn meal prepping into a habit, making it a regular part of your routine.

11. Embrace Leftovers:

Cook once, eat twice. Plan for meals that will give you leftovers, which can be used for lunches or repurposed into a new meal the next day.

12. Freeze for Later: If you make a large batch of a meal, freeze portions for later. This can be a lifesaver during particularly busy times when you might not be able to prep.

13. Keep It Simple: Not every meal has to be a culinary masterpiece. Simple meals can be nutritious and align with the DASH diet principles. Don't overcomplicate your meal prep.

14. Record Your Favorites: Keep a record of meal prep recipes that you enjoy and that fit well within the DASH diet. This makes planning easier and helps to build a repertoire of go-to meals.

15. Stay Flexible: Life can be unpredictable, so it's important to stay flexible with your meal prep. If something doesn't go as planned, adjust your schedule or meal plan as needed.

28 Days Structured Meal Plan

Week 1

Day 1:

- Breakfast: Grilled Lemon Herb Chicken Salad
- Lunch: Turkey and Vegetable Stir-Fry leftovers
- Dinner: Quinoa Stuffed Bell Peppers
- Snacks: Fresh fruit, a handful of nuts

Day 2:

- Breakfast: Oatmeal with diced apples and cinnamon
- Lunch: Lentil Soup with Kale leftovers
- Dinner: Baked Salmon with Dill Yogurt Sauce
- Snacks: Veggie sticks with hummus

Day 3:

- Breakfast: Whole Wheat Toast with Avocado and Poached Egg
- Lunch: Grilled Lemon Herb Chicken Salad leftovers
- Dinner: Turkey and Vegetable Stir-Fry
- Snacks: Greek yogurt with berries

Day 4:

- Breakfast: Fruit and Yogurt Parfait
- Lunch: Quinoa Stuffed Bell Peppers leftovers
- Dinner: Lentil Soup with Kale
- Snacks: Whole grain crackers with cheese

Day 5:

- Breakfast: Smoothie with spinach, banana, and almond milk
- Lunch: Baked Salmon with Dill Yogurt Sauce leftovers
- Dinner: Whole Wheat Pasta with Tomato Basil Sauce
- Snacks: Apple slices with almond butter

Day 6:

- Breakfast: Scrambled Eggs with Spinach and Whole Wheat Toast
- Lunch: Lentil Soup with Kale leftovers
- Dinner: Veggie Fajitas with Black Beans
- Snacks: Cottage cheese with pineapple

Day 7:

- Breakfast: Oatmeal with mixed berries and chia seeds

- Lunch: Whole Wheat Pasta with Tomato Basil Sauce leftovers
- Dinner: Grilled Chicken with Steamed Vegetables
- Snacks: Raw nuts and dried fruit

Week 2

Day 8:

- Breakfast: Greek Yogurt with Granola and Honey
- Lunch: Veggie Fajitas with Black Beans leftovers
- Dinner: Quinoa Stuffed Bell Peppers
- Snacks: Carrot sticks with tzatziki

Day 9:

- Breakfast: Whole Grain Pancakes with Fresh Berries
- Lunch: Grilled Chicken Salad with Mixed Greens
- Dinner: Baked Salmon with Dill Yogurt Sauce
- Snacks: Banana and a handful of almonds

Day 10:

- Breakfast: Avocado Toast with Tomato Slices
- Lunch: Quinoa Stuffed Bell Peppers leftovers
- Dinner: Turkey and Vegetable Stir-Fry
- Snacks: Celery sticks with peanut butter

Day 11:

- Breakfast: Smoothie Bowl with Fresh Fruit and Nuts
- Lunch: Baked Salmon with Dill Yogurt Sauce leftovers
- Dinner: Lentil Soup with Kale
- Snacks: Cottage cheese with sliced peaches

Day 12:

- Breakfast: Scrambled Tofu with Spinach and Mushrooms
- Lunch: Turkey and Vegetable Stir-Fry leftovers
- Dinner: Whole Wheat Pasta with Tomato Basil Sauce
- Snacks: Fresh fruit salad

Day 13:

- Breakfast: Omelette with Peppers, Onions, and Low-Fat Cheese
- Lunch: Lentil Soup with Kale leftovers
- Dinner: Veggie Fajitas with Black Beans
- Snacks: Greek yogurt with a drizzle of honey

Day 14:

- Breakfast: Chia Seed Pudding with Mixed Berries

- Lunch: Whole Wheat Pasta with Tomato Basil Sauce leftovers
- Dinner: Grilled Fish with Quinoa and Steamed Broccoli
- Snacks: Sliced cucumber and cherry tomatoes

Week 3

Day 15:

- Breakfast: Berry and Banana Smoothie
- Lunch: Chickpea Salad with Mixed Greens
- Dinner: Grilled Turkey Burger with Sweet Potato Fries
- Snacks: Sliced bell peppers and hummus

Day 16:

- Breakfast: Whole Grain Cereal with Skim Milk and Strawberries
- Lunch: Tuna Salad on Whole Wheat Bread
- Dinner: Stir-Fried Tofu with Broccoli and Brown Rice
- Snacks: Greek yogurt with a sprinkle of nuts

Day 17:

- Breakfast: Egg White Omelet with Spinach and Mushrooms

79

- Lunch: Quinoa and Black Bean Salad
- Dinner: Baked Cod with Steamed Asparagus and Quinoa
- Snacks: Apple slices with peanut butter

Day 18:

- Breakfast: Whole Wheat Pancakes with Blueberries
- Lunch: Grilled Chicken Caesar Salad (low-fat dressing)
- Dinner: Vegetarian Chili
- Snacks: Carrot and cucumber sticks

Day 19:

- Breakfast: Oatmeal with Sliced Banana and Almonds
- Lunch: Turkey and Avocado Wrap
- Dinner: Lemon Garlic Shrimp with Zucchini Noodles
- Snacks: A handful of mixed nuts

Day 20:

- Breakfast: Greek Yogurt with Mixed Berries and Chia Seeds
- Lunch: Lentil and Vegetable Soup

- Dinner: Chicken Stir-Fry with Mixed Vegetables and Brown Rice
- Snacks: Fresh fruit salad

Day 21:

- Breakfast: Scrambled Eggs with Diced Tomatoes and Spinach
- Lunch: Caprese Salad with Whole Wheat Bread
- Dinner: Baked Trout with Roasted Brussels Sprouts
- Snacks: Cottage cheese with sliced pineapple

Week 4

Day 22:

- Breakfast: Protein Smoothie with Spinach, Banana, and Almond Milk
- Lunch: Mediterranean Quinoa Bowl
- Dinner: Grilled Chicken with Mixed Vegetable Kabobs
- Snacks: Sliced pear with a handful of almonds

Day 23:

- Breakfast: Whole Wheat Toast with Avocado and Tomato Slices

- Lunch: Spinach and Goat Cheese Salad with Grilled Chicken
- Dinner: Spaghetti Squash with Tomato Sauce and Meatballs
- Snacks: Celery sticks with almond butter

Day 24:

- Breakfast: Cottage Cheese with Fresh Peaches
- Lunch: Grilled Salmon Salad with Mixed Greens
- Dinner: Veggie Burger on Whole Wheat Bun with Side Salad
- Snacks: A small bowl of mixed berries

Day 25:

- Breakfast: Muesli with Skim Milk and Dried Fruit
- Lunch: Chicken and Vegetable Soup
- Dinner: Beef Stir-Fry with Broccoli and Brown Rice
- Snacks: Greek yogurt with honey

Day 26:

- Breakfast: Poached Eggs on Whole Grain Toast
- Lunch: Tuna Nicoise Salad
- Dinner: Roasted Chicken with Sweet Potatoes and Green Beans

- Snacks: A handful of raw vegetables with low-fat dip

Day 27:

- Breakfast: Fruit Salad with a Dollop of Greek Yogurt
- Lunch: Quinoa Stuffed Avocado
- Dinner: Pork Tenderloin with Roasted Carrots and Parsnips
- Snacks: Whole grain crackers with cheese

Day 28:

- Breakfast: Baked Oatmeal with Apples and Cinnamon
- Lunch: Roasted Beet and Goat Cheese Salad
- Dinner: Grilled Shrimp with Brown Rice Pilaf and Steamed Broccoli
- Snacks: A small handful of walnuts

CHAPTER 6

NAVIGATING DIETARY CHALLENGES

Navigating the dietary challenges of the DASH Diet is crucial for anyone looking to successfully implement and maintain this eating plan. While the DASH Diet is renowned for its health benefits, particularly in reducing hypertension and aiding in weight loss, adhering to it can present certain challenges. These include dining out, handling cravings, and adapting the diet to meet unique dietary requirements. Addressing these challenges effectively is key to making the DASH Diet a sustainable part of one's lifestyle.

Strategies for Dining Out:

Dining out can be one of the more significant challenges when following the DASH Diet, as restaurant meals often contain higher levels of sodium and unhealthy fats. However, with a strategic approach, you can enjoy dining out without derailing your diet plan.

- **Menu Research:** Before visiting a restaurant, research their menu online. Many restaurants provide nutritional information, allowing you to make informed choices that align with the DASH Diet's guidelines.

- **Communicate with the Staff:** Don't hesitate to ask the serving staff about how dishes are prepared. Request modifications if necessary, such as dressing on the side or grilled instead of fried options.

- **Mindful of Portions:** Restaurant portions can be significantly larger than recommended serving sizes. Consider sharing a dish or asking for a half portion. Alternatively, you could immediately box half of your meal to take home.

- **Choose Wisely:** Opt for dishes rich in vegetables, whole grains, and lean proteins. Avoid items described as creamy, breaded, battered, or fried, as these are likely high in unhealthy fats and sodium.

- **Limiting Sodium:** Ask for your dish to be prepared with less salt, and avoid adding extra salt at the table. Also, be cautious with condiments like soy sauce or ketchup, which can be high in sodium.

Handling Cravings:

Cravings, especially for foods high in salt, sugar, or unhealthy fats, can be a significant hurdle in maintaining the DASH Diet.

Healthy Substitutes: Find healthier alternatives that satisfy your cravings. For instance, if you crave something sweet, opt for fresh fruit or a small piece of dark chocolate instead of sugary processed snacks.

Stay Hydrated: Sometimes, what feels like a craving is actually thirst. Drinking water or herbal tea can help mitigate these false hunger signals.

Mindful Eating: Pay attention to your eating habits. Eating slowly and without distractions can help you recognize when you're truly hungry and when you're eating out of habit or emotion.

Plan Your Meals and Snacks: Having a plan for your meals and snacks can help prevent impulsive eating.

Prepare healthy snacks in advance so you have them on hand when cravings strike.

Understand Your Cravings: Sometimes cravings can be linked to emotional needs. Understanding the root cause of your cravings can help you address them more effectively.

Adapting the DASH Diet for Unique Dietary Requirements

1. Vegetarian and Vegan Adaptations:

For vegetarians and vegans, the DASH Diet can be easily adapted by substituting animal proteins with plant-based sources. This adaptation not only aligns with the diet's emphasis on fruits, vegetables, and whole grains but also enhances its heart-healthy benefits.

- **Protein Sources:** Beans, lentils, tofu, tempeh, and edamame are excellent sources of plant-based protein. Nuts and seeds, including chia, flaxseeds, and hemp seeds, can also be incorporated for added protein and other nutrients.
- **Nutrient Considerations:** Pay attention to nutrients that may be less abundant in a plant-

based diet, such as iron, calcium, vitamin B12, and omega-3 fatty acids. Fortified plant-based milks and cereals can help address these needs.

- **Diverse Plant-Based Meals:** Embrace a variety of fruits, vegetables, whole grains, and legumes to ensure a wide range of nutrients. Experiment with different herbs and spices for flavor without adding excess sodium.

2. Gluten-Free Needs:

Individuals with celiac disease or gluten sensitivity can follow the DASH Diet by choosing gluten-free whole grains and being mindful of processed foods.

- **Gluten-Free Grains:** Brown rice, quinoa, buckwheat, millet, and gluten-free oats are excellent choices. These grains provide the fiber and nutrients integral to the DASH Diet without the gluten.
- **Reading Labels:** Be vigilant about reading food labels, as gluten can be present in unexpected products. Watch out for processed foods that might use gluten-containing ingredients.

- **Whole Foods Focus:** Emphasize naturally gluten-free whole foods like fruits, vegetables, lean proteins, and dairy or dairy alternatives.

3. Lactose Intolerance:

For those who are lactose intolerant, the DASH Diet's dairy component can be modified without losing the nutritional benefits.

- **Lactose-Free Dairy Products:** Many stores offer lactose-free versions of milk, yogurt, and cheese. These products provide the same nutrients as their lactose-containing counterparts.
- **Plant-Based Alternatives:** Almond, soy, oat, and rice milks are viable alternatives. Choose unsweetened versions and check for fortification with calcium and vitamin D.
- **Calcium-Rich Foods:** Incorporate other calcium-rich foods like leafy green vegetables, almonds, tofu, and fortified foods to meet calcium needs.

4. Low-Carb Considerations:

While the DASH Diet includes whole grains, it can be adapted for those seeking a lower-carb approach.

- **Reducing Grains:** You can reduce the grain portion sizes and increase non-starchy vegetables and lean proteins.
- **Low-Carb Vegetables:** Focus on vegetables that are low in carbohydrates, such as leafy greens, peppers, cucumbers, and zucchini.
- **Healthy Fats:** Include sources of healthy fats like avocados, nuts, and seeds to maintain satiety.

5. Allergies and Food Intolerances:

Individual food allergies and intolerances require specific modifications to the DASH Diet.

- **Substitute Wisely:** For any allergen, find nutritionally equivalent substitutes. For example, if you're allergic to nuts, seeds might be a suitable alternative.
- **Consult a Dietitian:** If you have multiple food allergies or complex dietary needs, consulting with a dietitian can help ensure that your modified DASH Diet is nutritionally balanced.

CHAPTER 7

PHYSICAL ACTIVITY AND THE DASH DIET

Exercise-Diet Synergy

The synergy between the DASH Diet and regular physical activity is a cornerstone of a holistic approach to health and wellness. This powerful combination not only enhances cardiovascular health and aids in weight management but also improves metabolic health and mental well-being. Let's delve deeper into each of these aspects to understand how this synergy works and its profound benefits.

Enhanced Cardiovascular Health

Cardiovascular health is paramount for overall well-being, and the combination of the DASH Diet and regular exercise plays a significant role in its improvement. The DASH Diet, with its emphasis on fruits, vegetables, whole grains, and lean proteins, provides essential nutrients like potassium and magnesium, which are known for their heart health benefits.

- **Role of Nutrients in Cardiovascular Health:** Potassium helps regulate heart function and blood pressure by balancing out the negative effects of salt. Magnesium, on the other hand, aids in maintaining a healthy heartbeat and is crucial in converting food into energy. When these nutrients are combined with a regular exercise regimen, they work together to strengthen the heart muscle, improve blood flow, and reduce the risk of heart diseases.

- **Impact of Exercise on Heart Health:** Regular physical activity, especially aerobic exercises like walking, jogging, and cycling, increases the heart rate and improves its efficiency in pumping blood. This not only helps in lowering blood pressure but also reduces the strain on the heart. Over time, this can lead to a significant decrease in the risk of heart diseases, including heart attacks and strokes.

- **Combining Diet and Exercise for Optimal Heart Health:** By following the DASH Diet and engaging in regular physical activity, individuals can create a comprehensive approach to heart health. This combination not only provides the body with the necessary nutrients to support heart function but also strengthens the heart through physical activity.

Weight Management

Managing weight effectively is a common challenge, but the combination of the DASH Diet and exercise offers a balanced approach to achieving and maintaining a healthy weight.

- **Caloric Balance and Weight Loss:** The DASH Diet focuses on low-calorie, nutrient-rich foods, which naturally leads to a reduction in overall caloric intake. When this is paired with the calorie-burning effects of exercise, it creates a caloric deficit, which is essential for weight loss.

- **Exercise and Energy Expenditure:** Regular physical activity increases the body's energy expenditure. Activities like strength training build muscle mass, which in turn increases the resting metabolic rate, meaning more calories are burned even when at rest. Aerobic exercises, such as running or swimming, burn calories during the activity, contributing directly to weight loss.

- **Sustainable Weight Management:** The key to successful weight management is sustainability. The DASH Diet, being rich in fruits, vegetables, and whole grains, is not only nutritious but also satiating, making it easier to stick to in the long term. When combined with a regular exercise routine, it forms a sustainable lifestyle change rather than a short-term diet, leading to long-term weight management.

Improved Metabolic Health

Metabolic health is another crucial aspect of overall wellness, and the synergy between the DASH Diet and exercise significantly contributes to its improvement.

- **Regulation of Blood Sugar Levels:** Regular physical activity improves insulin sensitivity, which is crucial for the regulation of blood sugar levels. This is particularly beneficial for individuals following the DASH Diet, which is low in sugar and high in fiber. Fiber helps slow down the absorption of sugar in the bloodstream, preventing spikes in blood sugar levels.

- **Prevention and Management of Diabetes:** By improving insulin sensitivity and regulating blood sugar levels, the combination of the DASH Diet and regular exercise can play a significant role in the prevention and management of diabetes. This is especially important given the rising prevalence of diabetes globally.

- **Overall Metabolic Function:** Regular exercise and a balanced diet like the DASH Diet improve overall metabolic function. This includes better regulation of cholesterol levels, improved blood sugar control, and enhanced processing of fats in the body, all of which contribute to metabolic health.

Mental Health Benefits

The mental health benefits of combining the DASH Diet with regular exercise are often overlooked but are equally important.

- **Release of Endorphins:** Exercise is known to stimulate the release of endorphins, the body's natural mood elevators. This can lead to an improvement in mood and a reduction in feelings of depression and anxiety.

- **Stress Reduction:** Regular physical activity is an effective stress reliever. It provides a mental break from daily stressors and can improve sleep quality, which is crucial for mental health. The DASH Diet, with its balanced approach to nutrition, can also help stabilize mood and reduce stress levels.

- **Improved Cognitive Function:** There is growing evidence that regular physical activity, coupled with a healthy diet like the DASH Diet, can improve cognitive function and may reduce the risk of cognitive decline with age.

Recommended Exercises

Aerobic Exercises

Aerobic exercises, also known as cardio exercises, are crucial for improving cardiovascular health. These activities increase the heart rate and breathing, strengthening the heart and improving the efficiency of the circulatory system. Regular aerobic exercise can help lower blood pressure, a key goal of the DASH Diet, and reduce the risk of many chronic diseases.

I. **Walking:** Perhaps the most accessible form of exercise, walking can be easily incorporated into daily routines. It's low-impact, requires no special equipment, and can be done anywhere. A brisk walk for 30 minutes a day can significantly improve cardiovascular health.

II. **Jogging and Running:** These are more intense forms of aerobic exercise and are excellent for heart health. They can be more demanding on the joints, so it's important to have proper footwear and to start slowly, gradually increasing intensity and duration.

III. **Cycling:** Whether outdoor or indoor, cycling is a great low-impact aerobic exercise. It's effective for increasing heart rate and improving leg strength and endurance.

IV. **Swimming:** Swimming is a full-body workout that combines cardiovascular exercise with muscle strengthening. It's particularly beneficial for those with joint issues or arthritis, as it's a low-impact activity.

V. **Dancing:** Dancing is not only a fun way to stay active but also an effective aerobic workout. It can vary in intensity and often involves learning routines, which can also benefit cognitive health.

Strength Training

Strength training, or resistance training, involves exercises that improve muscle strength and endurance. This type of exercise is important for overall health, as it helps build lean muscle mass, which can increase metabolic rate and aid in weight loss.

I. **Weight Lifting:** This can be done with free weights, weight machines, or even body weight. Exercises like squats, lunges, and bench presses are effective for building strength. It's important to focus on form to prevent injuries.

II. **Resistance Bands:** These are a versatile and low-cost option for strength training. They come in various resistance levels and can be used for a full-body workout.

III. **Bodyweight Exercises:** Push-ups, sit-ups, and planks are examples of exercises that use body weight for resistance. They can be done anywhere and are effective for building strength.

Flexibility and Balance Exercises

Flexibility and balance exercises are often overlooked but are crucial for overall fitness and injury prevention. They improve muscle elasticity, joint mobility, and balance, which are important for everyday activities.

I. **Yoga:** Yoga combines physical postures, breathing exercises, and meditation. It improves flexibility, balance, and muscle tone. Yoga also offers mental health benefits, reducing stress and anxiety.

II. **Pilates:** Pilates focuses on core strength, flexibility, and overall body awareness. It involves precise movements and breathing techniques and is excellent for improving posture and balance.

III. **Stretching:** Regular stretching is important for maintaining flexibility. It can be done as a part of a warm-up or cool-down during workouts or as a standalone activity.

High-Intensity Interval Training (HIIT)

HIIT involves short bursts of intense exercise followed by periods of rest or lower-intensity exercise. It's a time-efficient way to combine aerobic and strength exercises and has been shown to improve cardiovascular fitness, strength, and metabolic health.

I. **Circuit Training:** This involves a series of exercises performed one after the other with minimal rest in between. It can combine aerobic exercises like jumping jacks with strength exercises like squats.

II. **Tabata Training:** A form of HIIT, Tabata involves 20 seconds of intense effort followed by 10 seconds of rest, repeated eight times. It's a quick and effective workout that can be done in under 30 minutes.

III. **Sprint Intervals:** Alternating between sprints and walking or jogging is a simple form of HIIT that can be done outdoors or on a treadmill.

Tailoring Your Exercise Regimen

1. Assess Fitness Level:

Understanding your current fitness level is the foundation of creating an effective exercise plan. This assessment should consider various aspects:

- **Stamina:** Evaluate how long you can engage in physical activities like walking, jogging, or swimming before feeling exhausted. This gives an indication of your cardiovascular health.
- **Strength:** Assess your muscle strength. Can you carry groceries easily? How many push-ups or squats can you do? This helps in determining the starting point for strength training.
- **Flexibility:** Check how flexible you are. Can you touch your toes without bending your knees? Flexibility is crucial for preventing injuries.
- **Balance:** Balance exercises are often overlooked but are essential, especially as we age.

2. Consider Health Conditions:

If you have health conditions, particularly those related to heart health like hypertension, it's imperative to consult with a healthcare provider. They can provide guidance on safe exercise limits and recommend types of exercises that are beneficial and those to avoid. For instance, someone with high blood pressure might be advised to avoid heavy weightlifting.

3. Set Realistic Goals:

Setting achievable goals is crucial. These should be based on your fitness assessment and health considerations. Goals can be short-term (like walking 30 minutes a day) or long-term (like running a 5K). Remember:

- **Start Slow:** If you're new to exercising, begin with low-intensity activities and gradually increase the intensity.
- **SMART Goals:** Ensure your goals are Specific, Measurable, Achievable, Relevant, and Time-bound.

4. Choose Enjoyable Activities:

Enjoyment is key to maintaining an exercise routine. If you enjoy what you're doing, you're more likely to stick with it. This could mean:

- **Outdoor Activities:** If you love nature, consider hiking, cycling, or jogging in the park.
- **Group Classes:** For those who thrive in social settings, group classes like Zumba or spinning might be appealing.

- **Home Workouts:** If you prefer privacy, home workout videos or equipment might be more suitable.

5. Incorporate Variety:

Variety not only keeps boredom at bay but also ensures that different muscle groups are engaged, and various fitness components are addressed. This could include:

- **Mixing Cardio and Strength:** Balance cardio exercises like running with strength training exercises like weightlifting.
- **Trying New Activities:** Experiment with different activities like yoga, Pilates, or martial arts.
- **Seasonal Changes:** Adapt your activities to the seasons – swimming in summer, skiing in winter, for instance.

6. Monitor Progress:

Tracking your progress is essential for motivation and for assessing the effectiveness of your exercise plan. This can be done through:

- **Fitness Apps:** Use apps to track your daily activities, steps, and workouts.

- **Journaling:** Keep an exercise diary to note down your workouts and how you feel after each session.
- **Fitness Trackers:** Wearable devices can monitor your heart rate, sleep patterns, and activity levels.

7. Align Exercise with Dietary Goals:

Your exercise routine should complement your dietary goals as per the DASH Diet. This involves:

- **Balancing Nutrient Intake:** On days of intense workouts, increase your protein intake for muscle repair. Also, ensure you're getting enough carbohydrates for energy.
- **Hydration:** Stay well-hydrated, especially before, during, and after workouts.
- **Post-Workout Meals:** Consume a balanced meal after exercising to replenish energy stores and aid in recovery.

8. Stay Consistent:

Consistency is the key to reaping long-term benefits. To maintain regular physical activity:

- **Set a Schedule:** Try to exercise at the same time each day to establish a routine.

- **Be Flexible:** If you miss a workout, don't get discouraged. Adjust as needed and get back on track.

- **Listen to Your Body:** Rest when needed. Overtraining can lead to burnout and injuries.

CHAPTER 8

LIFESTYLE INTEGRATION

Stress Reduction Techniques

Stress is an inevitable part of life, but its management is crucial for maintaining both physical and mental health. The DASH Diet can be a tool in stress management, not just through the foods consumed but also through the lifestyle it promotes.

Mindful Eating: The DASH Diet encourages mindful eating, which involves being fully present and aware during meals. This practice can turn eating into a stress-reducing activity. Mindful eating helps in recognizing hunger and fullness cues, leading to a more satisfying and less stressful eating experience.

Balanced Nutrition: The diet's emphasis on fruits, vegetables, whole grains, and lean proteins ensures that the body gets a balanced mix of nutrients. Nutrients like omega-3 fatty acids, found in fish, have been shown to reduce the levels of stress hormones in the body. Magnesium, found in nuts and leafy greens, can help mitigate the body's stress response.

Regular Meal Times: Having structured meal times, as recommended by the DASH Diet, can provide a sense of routine and stability, which is beneficial in managing stress. Regular eating schedules prevent blood sugar dips, which can exacerbate stress and anxiety.

Diet's Impact on Mental Health

The connection between diet and mental health is a growing area of interest in the medical community. The DASH Diet, with its focus on heart health, inadvertently offers several benefits for mental health.

Brain Health: Foods rich in antioxidants, vitamins, and minerals, which are staples in the DASH Diet, are beneficial for brain health. For instance, antioxidants found in berries and leafy greens can help reduce inflammation and oxidative stress, which are linked to mental health disorders.

Gut-Brain Axis: There is increasing evidence supporting the gut-brain axis, where the health of the gut influences mental health. The high fiber content in the DASH Diet supports gut health, which in turn can positively impact mood and cognitive functions.

Blood Sugar Regulation: The DASH Diet's low sugar and high fiber content help in maintaining stable blood sugar levels. Fluctuations in blood sugar can impact mood and energy levels, contributing to symptoms of anxiety and depression.

Cultivating Community Support

Adopting a diet like the DASH Diet can be more sustainable and enjoyable when there is a sense of community support.

Sharing Meals: Preparing and sharing DASH-friendly meals can be a way to build community and support. It creates an opportunity for social interaction, which is vital for mental health.

Support Groups: Joining support groups, either in-person or online, where members follow the DASH Diet can provide a platform for sharing experiences, challenges, and successes. This communal support can be motivating and reassuring.

Educational Workshops: Participating in workshops or cooking classes focused on the DASH Diet can enhance knowledge and skills while providing an avenue to meet others with similar health and dietary goals.

Understanding the Importance of Monitoring Health Improvements

Monitoring health improvements is vital in any health and wellness journey. It provides tangible evidence of progress, helps in maintaining motivation, and allows for adjustments to be made to the diet or lifestyle as needed. For those following the DASH Diet, monitoring not only encompasses weight loss but also includes tracking changes in blood pressure, cholesterol levels, and overall physical and mental well-being.

Digital Tools for Health Tracking

In the digital age, numerous tools have emerged to aid individuals in tracking their health improvements. These tools range from simple mobile apps to sophisticated wearable devices. They offer a convenient and efficient way to record and analyze various health parameters.

Mobile Health Apps: There are numerous mobile applications designed for health tracking. These apps can track dietary intake, physical activity, and even sleep patterns. Many of them are tailored to specific diets or health goals and can be a great asset for those following the DASH Diet. They often include features like barcode scanners for logging food items, databases of nutritional information, and tools for setting and tracking personal health goals.

Wearable Devices: Wearable technology like fitness trackers and smartwatches has revolutionized personal health monitoring. These devices continuously track physical activity, heart rate, sleep quality, and sometimes even blood pressure and blood glucose levels. They sync with smartphones or computers, providing real-time data and long-term trends in health metrics.

Online Health Portals: Many healthcare providers now offer online portals where patients can access their medical records, including test results and health metrics. These portals often allow patients to track changes over time and can be a valuable resource for understanding the broader picture of one's health.

Interpreting Health Metrics

While collecting data is important, understanding what this data means is crucial for it to be useful. Interpreting health metrics involves looking at the numbers in the context of individual health goals and the specific parameters of the DASH Diet.

Blood Pressure Readings: Since the DASH Diet is particularly effective in managing hypertension, regular monitoring of blood pressure is essential. Understanding both systolic and diastolic numbers and how they align with healthy ranges is key. A decrease in these numbers often indicates success with the diet.

Weight and Body Mass Index (BMI): Tracking weight loss is more than just watching the scale. Understanding BMI and how it correlates with healthy body weight is important. However, it's also crucial to consider other factors like muscle mass and overall body composition.

Cholesterol Levels: The DASH Diet is known to positively impact cholesterol levels. Regular testing and understanding the difference between LDL (bad cholesterol) and HDL (good cholesterol) levels can provide insights into the effectiveness of the diet.

Dietary Intake: Monitoring what one eats is fundamental in the DASH Diet. This includes not just caloric intake but also the balance of nutrients like sodium, potassium, calcium, and fiber. Digital tools can help track these metrics and ensure adherence to the diet's guidelines.

Physical Activity Levels: Regular physical activity is a cornerstone of good health. Tracking exercise frequency, intensity, and type is important. Many digital tools provide insights into how physical activity impacts overall health and aids in achieving specific health goals.

Sleep Patterns: Good quality sleep is essential for health and well-being. Tracking sleep patterns can help identify issues like sleep apnea, which is often associated with hypertension and other health problems.

Mental Health: Mental well-being is just as important as physical health. Some digital tools offer features for tracking mood and stress levels, which can be particularly useful for understanding the holistic impact of the DASH Diet on one's life.

The Role of Healthcare Professionals

While digital tools provide valuable data, the role of healthcare professionals in interpreting this data cannot be overstated. Regular check-ups and discussions about the data collected with a healthcare provider can provide deeper insights and help tailor the DASH Diet and other lifestyle interventions more effectively.

Challenges and Considerations

While digital health tracking is beneficial, there are challenges and considerations to keep in mind. Data accuracy, privacy concerns, and the potential for becoming overly fixated on numbers are some of the issues that users should be aware of. It's also important to remember that these tools are aids in a health journey and not replacements for professional medical advice.

CHAPTER 9

ADVANCED WEIGHT LOSS TACTICS

Embarking on a weight loss journey often starts with basic dietary changes and increased physical activity. However, as one progresses, exploring advanced strategies can be beneficial in overcoming plateaus and achieving long-term success. Among these strategies, combining intermittent fasting with the DASH Diet, understanding the role of supplements, and sustaining weight loss and wellness are pivotal.

Combining Intermittent Fasting with the DASH Diet

Integrating Fasting and DASH Diet

Intermittent fasting (IF) is a dietary approach that cycles between periods of fasting and eating. It doesn't specify which foods to eat but rather when you should eat them. The most popular methods include the 16/8 method, where you fast for 16 hours and eat during an 8-hour window, and the 5:2 method, where you consume only 500-600 calories on two non-consecutive days of the week.

Combining IF with the DASH Diet can be a powerful tool. The DASH Diet, rich in fruits, vegetables, whole grains, and lean proteins, provides balanced nutrition. When paired with IF, it can enhance weight loss and health benefits. This combination works by not only reducing overall calorie intake but also by optimizing the timing of nutrient intake, which can have metabolic benefits.

Benefits and Precautions

The benefits of combining IF with the DASH Diet include improved metabolic health, potential weight loss, better blood sugar control, and reduced inflammation. However, precautions are necessary. IF is not suitable for everyone, especially those with certain health conditions like diabetes, or for pregnant or breastfeeding women. It's crucial to consult with a healthcare provider before starting IF, particularly when combining it with a specific diet like DASH.

Supplements and the DASH Diet

Indications for Supplements

While the DASH Diet is nutritionally comprehensive, certain individuals might require supplements to meet their specific health needs. For instance, someone with a vitamin D deficiency might need a supplement, especially if they have limited sun exposure or dietary intake of the vitamin.

Selecting Appropriate Supplements

Choosing the right supplements involves understanding one's unique nutritional needs and consulting with a healthcare provider. Common supplements that might be considered include vitamin D, omega-3 fatty acids, and calcium, especially for individuals who might not get enough from their diet.

Pros and Cons of Supplementation

Supplementation can help fill nutritional gaps, but it's not without drawbacks. Over-supplementation can lead to adverse effects, and some supplements might interact with medications. The key is to use supplements judiciously and under medical guidance, ensuring they complement the DASH Diet rather than replace its core principles of healthy eating.

Sustaining Weight Loss and Wellness

Keeping Weight Off Long-Term

Long-term weight maintenance is often more challenging than losing weight. It requires a sustainable approach to diet and lifestyle changes. The DASH Diet, with its focus on balanced eating and whole foods, is well-suited for long-term adherence. It's not a quick-fix diet but a lifestyle change that promotes overall health.

The DASH Diet as a Permanent Lifestyle

Adopting the DASH Diet as a permanent lifestyle involves more than just following a set of dietary guidelines. It's about creating a healthy relationship with food, understanding the importance of portion control, and enjoying a variety of nutrient-rich foods. It also means integrating regular physical activity into one's routine and making conscious choices about food.

Motivational Success Accounts

Success stories can be powerful motivators. Hearing about others who have successfully maintained their weight loss and improved their health on the DASH Diet can inspire and provide practical insights. These accounts often highlight the importance of consistency, the ability to overcome setbacks, and the integration of diet with overall lifestyle changes.

CONCLUSION

Our exploration of the DASH Diet as a weight loss solution has been extensive and multifaceted. We began with the inspiring story of Marsha Young from New Jersey, whose experience with the DASH Diet not only led to significant weight loss but also improved her overall health and lifestyle. Marsha's journey serves as a testament to the diet's effectiveness and its impact beyond just the numbers on the scale.

We delved into the key principles and health outcomes of the DASH Diet, highlighting its origins as a plan to combat hypertension and its evolution into a comprehensive dietary approach. The diet's emphasis on whole foods, lean proteins, and a balance of essential nutrients aligns with the fundamentals of healthy eating and weight management. Its focus on reducing processed foods, saturated fats, and sugar not only aids in weight loss but also contributes to overall health improvements, including better blood pressure and cholesterol levels.

The correlation between the DASH Diet and weight loss, while not the diet's primary intent, is significant. The diet's structure naturally leads to a reduction in calorie intake and promotes feelings of fullness, which are crucial for sustainable weight loss. Its emphasis on nutrient-rich foods and balanced meals supports long-term adherence, making it a viable option for those seeking not just to lose weight but to embrace a healthier lifestyle.

We also explored advanced weight loss tactics, including the integration of intermittent fasting with the DASH Diet, the role of supplements, and strategies for sustaining weight loss and wellness. Combining intermittent fasting with the DASH Diet can enhance weight loss and metabolic health, but it requires careful consideration and, in some cases, medical guidance. Supplements can be beneficial in filling nutritional gaps but should be used judiciously. Sustaining weight loss over the long term is perhaps the most challenging aspect, requiring a commitment to a permanent lifestyle change and a balanced approach to diet and exercise.

In essence, the DASH Diet is more than a dietary plan; it's a roadmap to a healthier, more balanced life. It offers a sustainable approach to eating that not only aids in weight loss but also improves overall health. The diet's flexibility, nutritional balance, and focus on whole foods make it adaptable and suitable for a wide range of individuals. Whether it's someone like Marsha Young looking to transform their health or anyone seeking a reliable and healthful dietary approach, the DASH Diet stands out as a comprehensive and effective solution.

Printed in Great Britain
by Amazon

34669990R00069